Meet Your Pelvic Floor:
What every woman should know

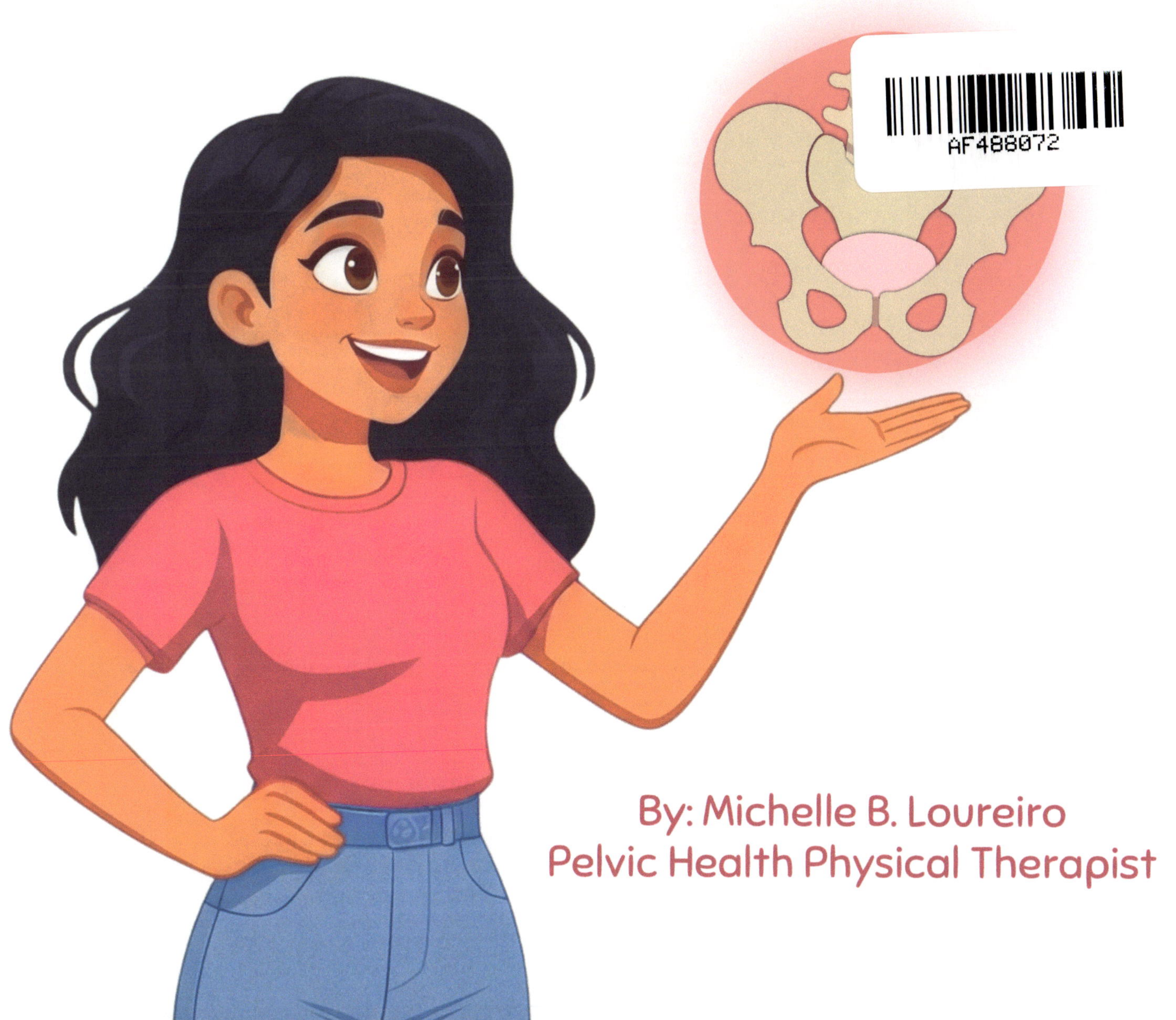

By: Michelle B. Loureiro
Pelvic Health Physical Therapist

Meet Your Pelvic Floor:
What every woman should know

Published by: Pelly & Co.
ISBN: 979-8-234-03571-4

*Disclaimer: The information in this book is for educational purposes only and is not
intended as medical advice. Please consult with a healthcare professional for your
specific needs.*

Dedication

To every woman who has ever wondered
or worried about her pelvic health...

May this book bring you knowledge,
reassurance, and confidence.

Let's continue to share this wisdom,
so that one day, we no longer hear:

"I wish I had known this sooner."

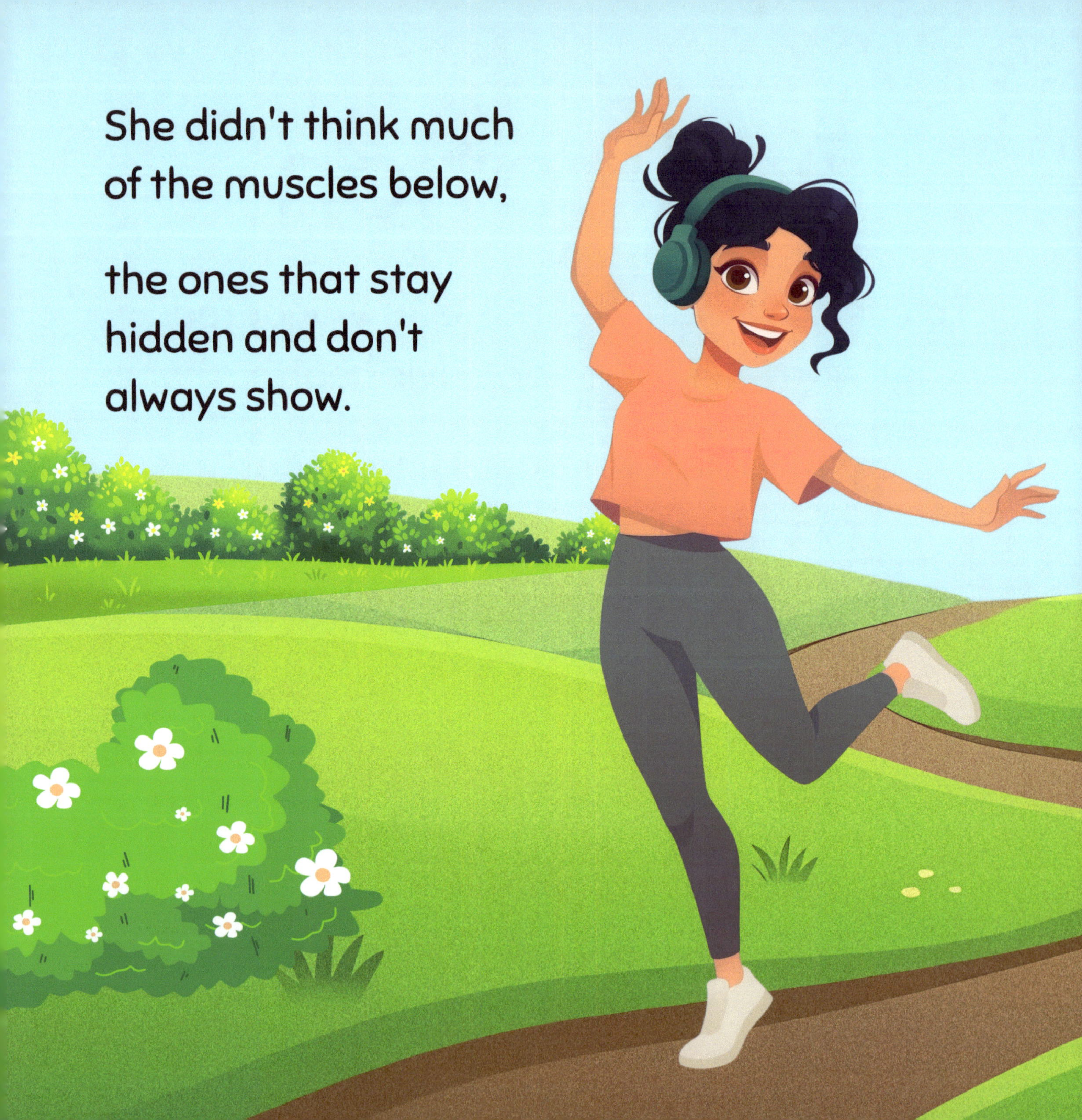

She didn't think much
of the muscles below,

the ones that stay
hidden and don't
always show.

She was busy with life, a heart light and free,
As happy and active as a person could be.

Through working and laughing, exercise and fun,
Her body carried her bravely until each day was done.

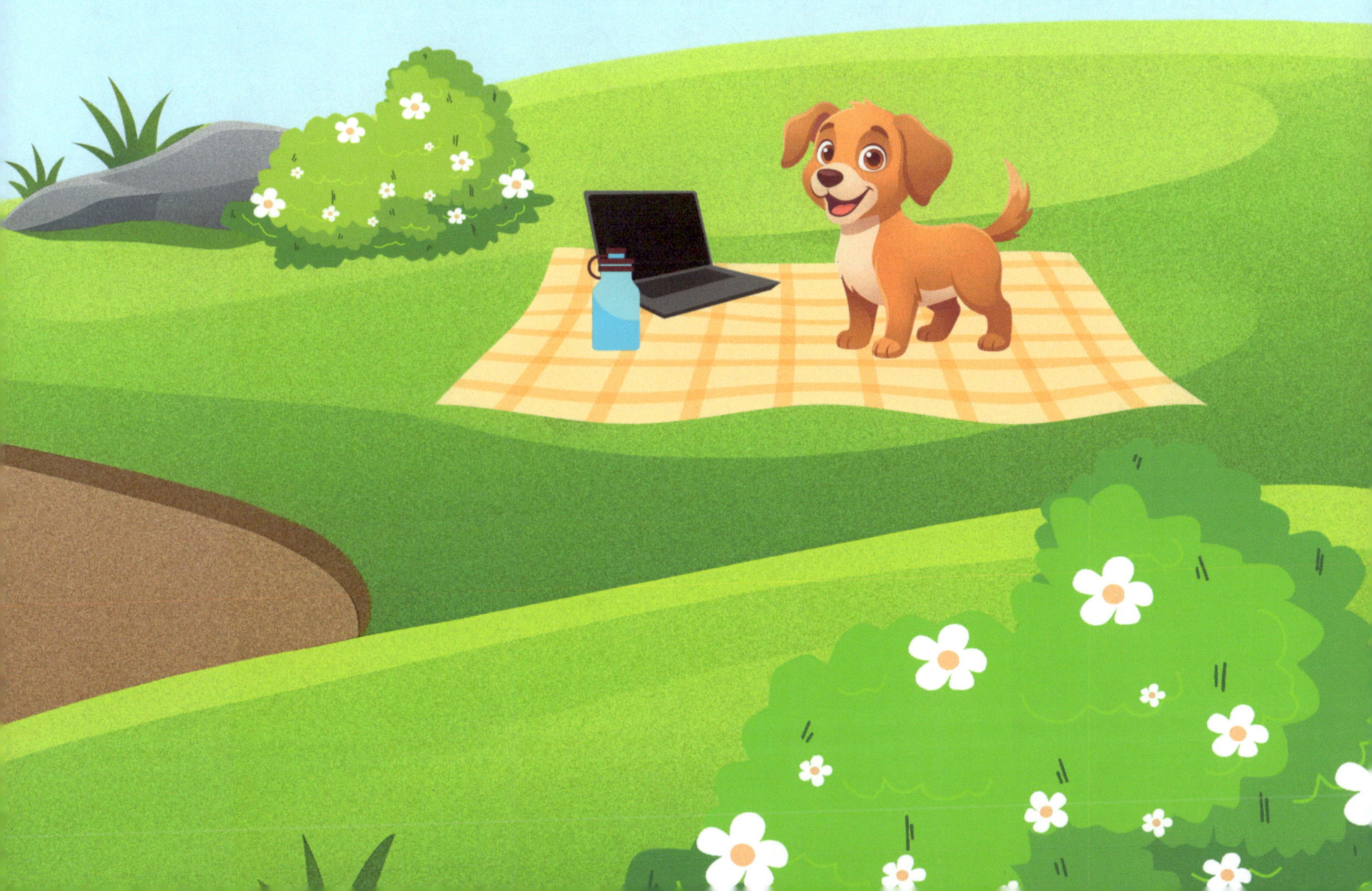

But then came a day,
with one great big laugh,
when her body took such
a surprising new path.

A moment, a startle,
a tiny surprise...
A small little leak
right before her own eyes.

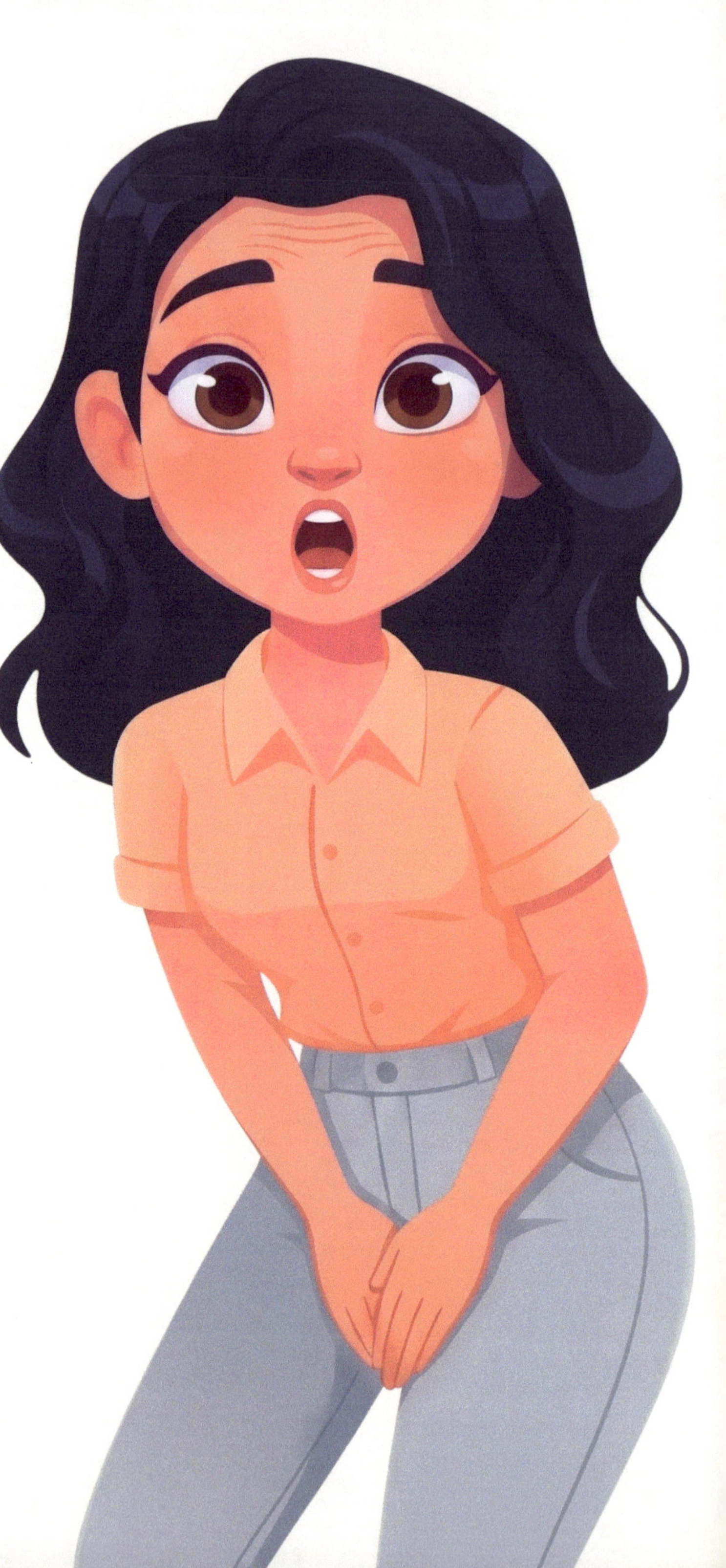

Other times, there was
heaviness, pressure, or pain.
An unwelcome new burden,
a strange kind of strain.

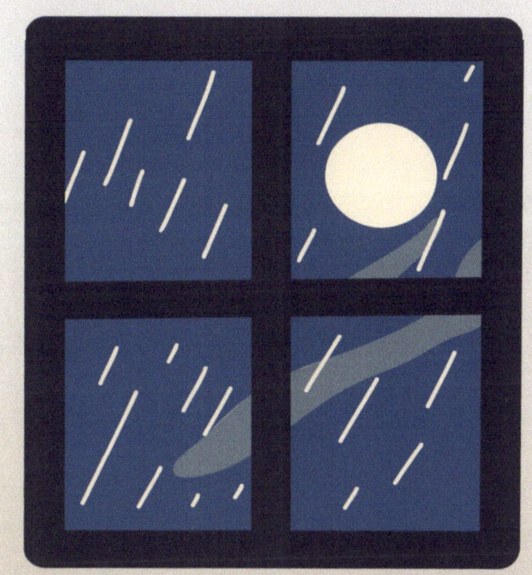

She wondered and worried,
and started to fear
"Is this my new normal?
Must I live with this here?"

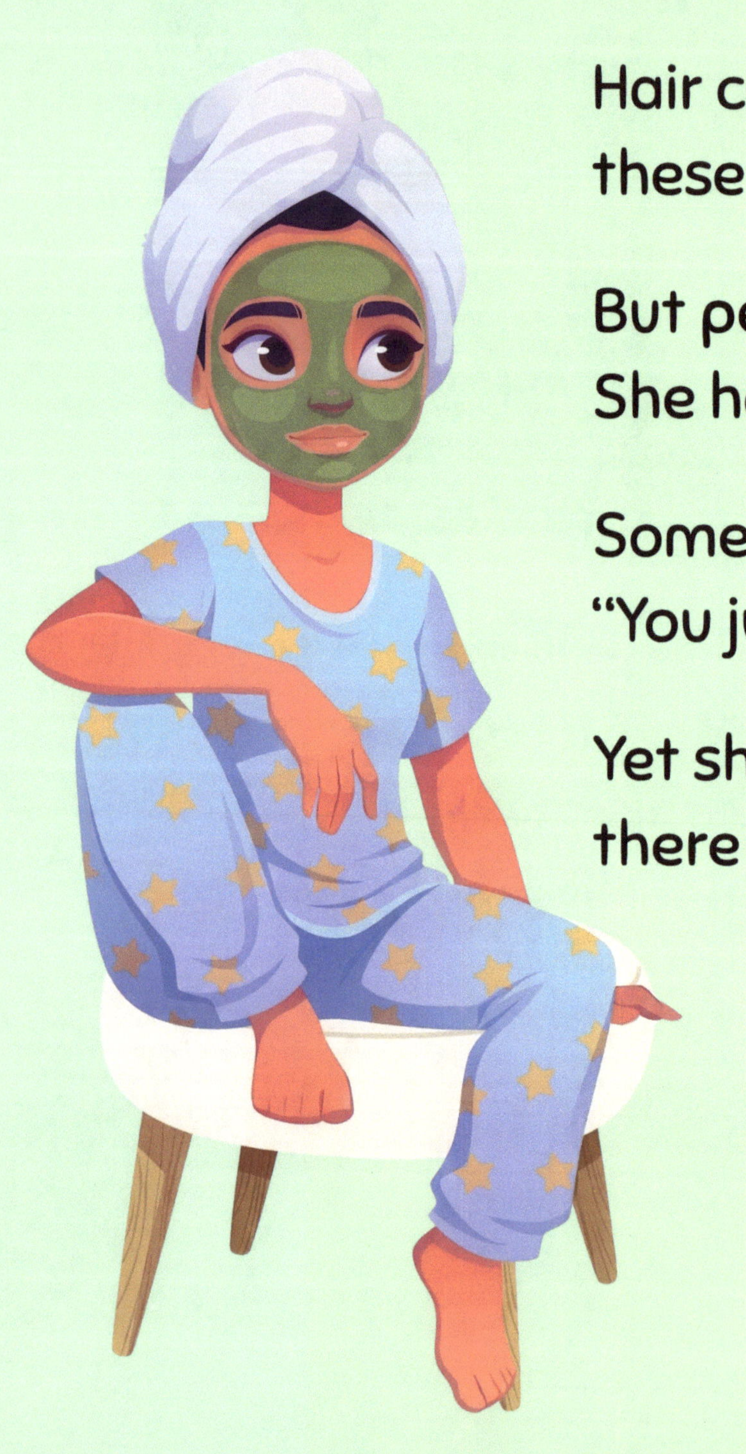

Hair care and skin care,
these things she knew.

But pelvic floor health?
She hadn't a clue.

Some said it was common...
"You just have to deal!"

Yet she knew in her heart,
there must be some way to heal.

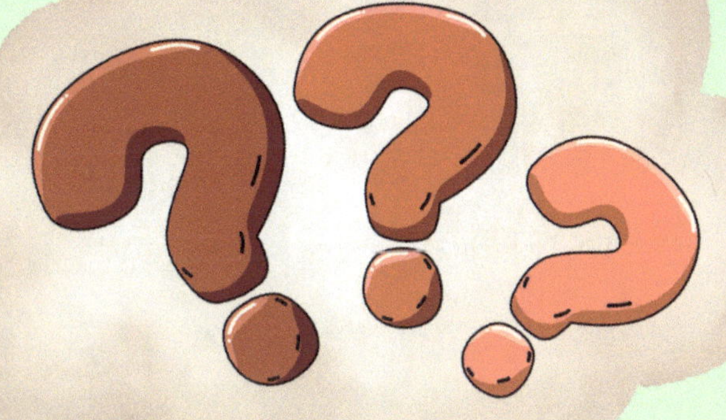

So she put to rest every concern and doubt,
to learn what the pelvic floor was really about.

She found the pelvic floor
was hidden deep down inside.
At the base of the pelvis
is where it would reside.

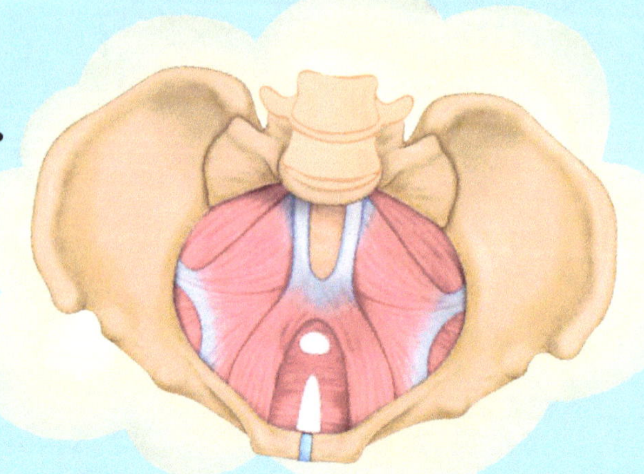

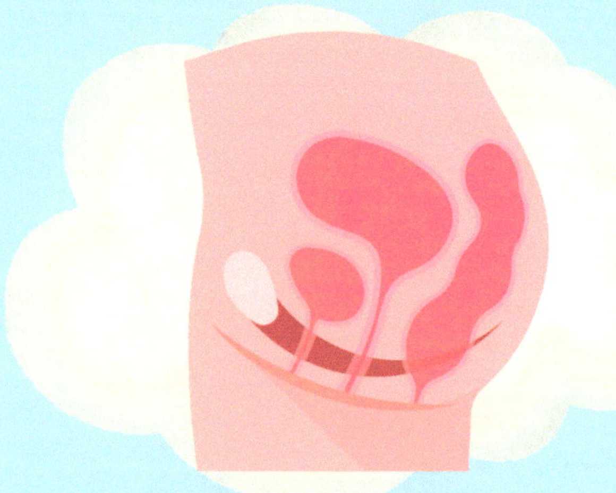

Shaped like a hammock,
both flexible and strong,
it's where all of the
pelvic organs belong.

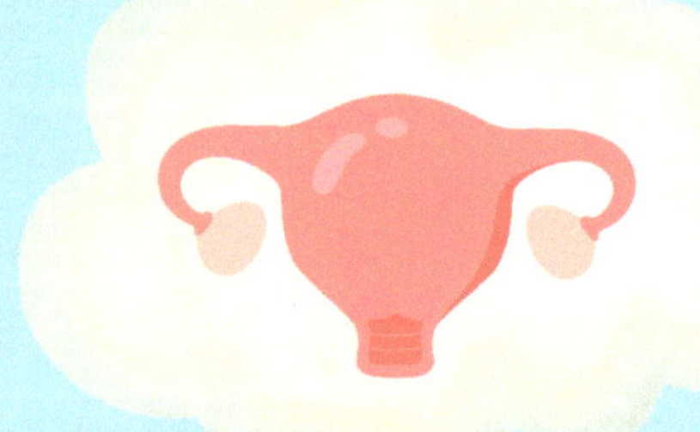

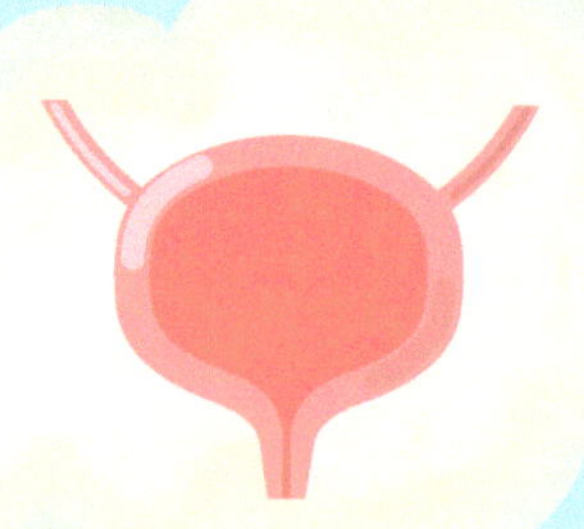

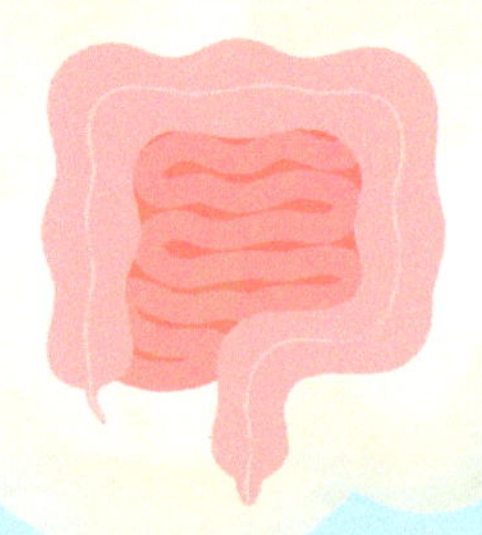

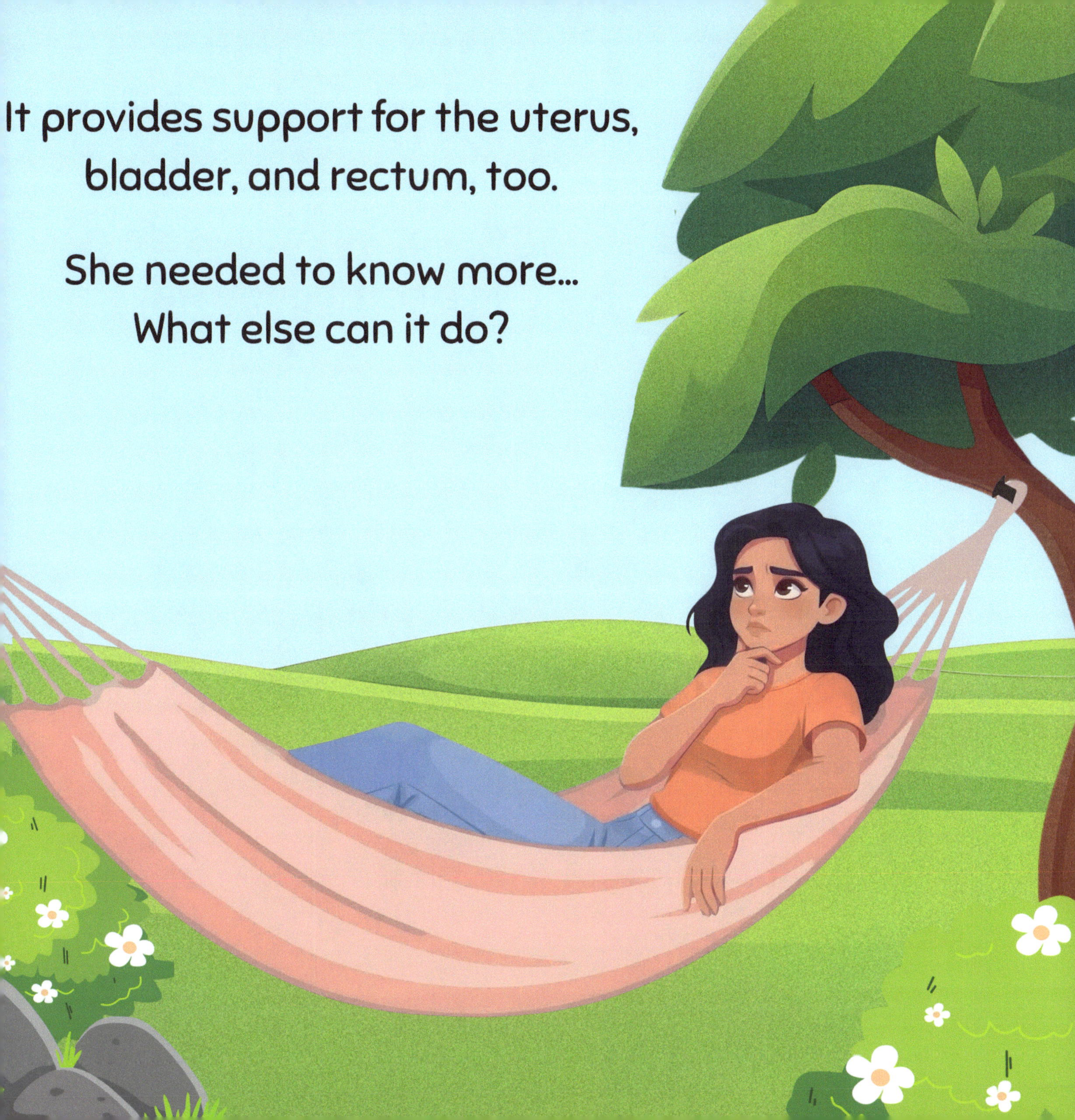

It provides support for the uterus,
bladder, and rectum, too.

She needed to know more...
What else can it do?

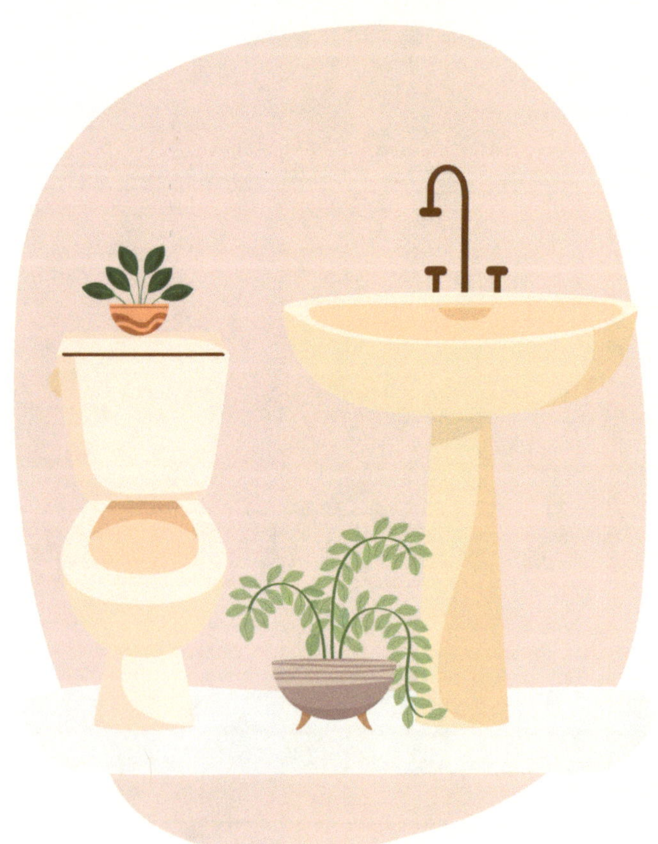

It aids both the bladder
and bowel each day.
Keeps intimacy safe
in a soft, gentle way.

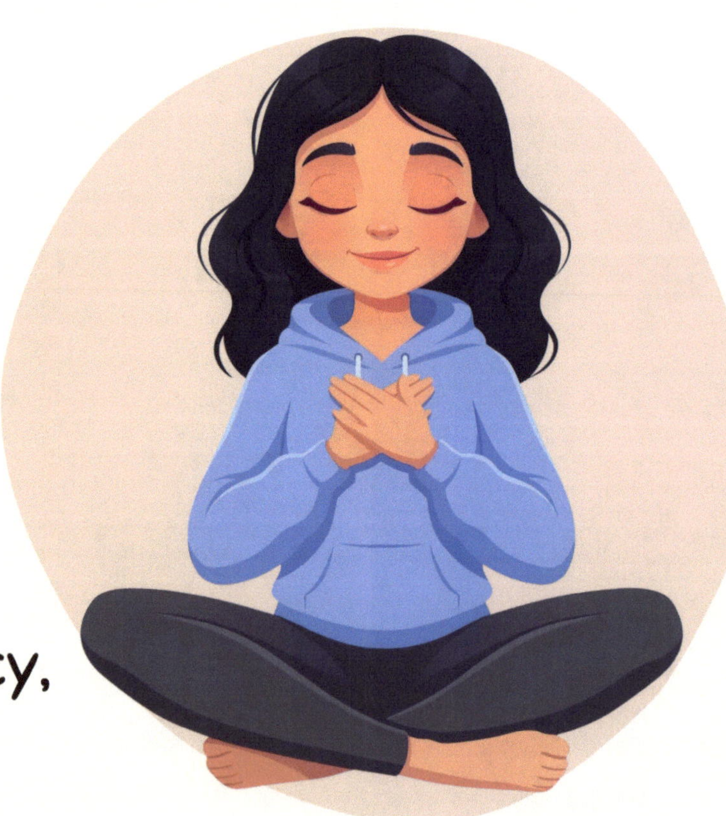

It moves with each breath
and steadies the core.
And lifts through pregnancy,
this strong pelvic floor.

And to her surprise, it's simply a muscle!
Like her arms and her legs, built for effort and hustle.

It contracts to lift and help her stay strong,
then softens and lengthens to move life along.

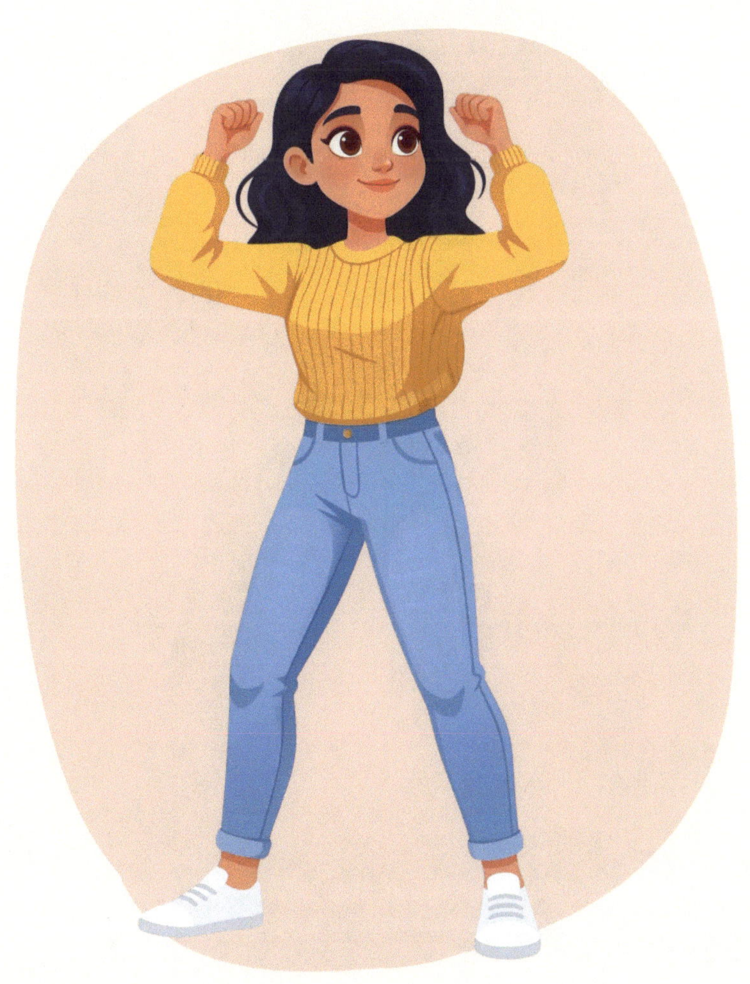

The bladder and bowel send it signals on cue,
it works in that moment, knows just what to do.

Like a stoplight shining a steady red glow,
"Not yet" is the message when it's not time to go.

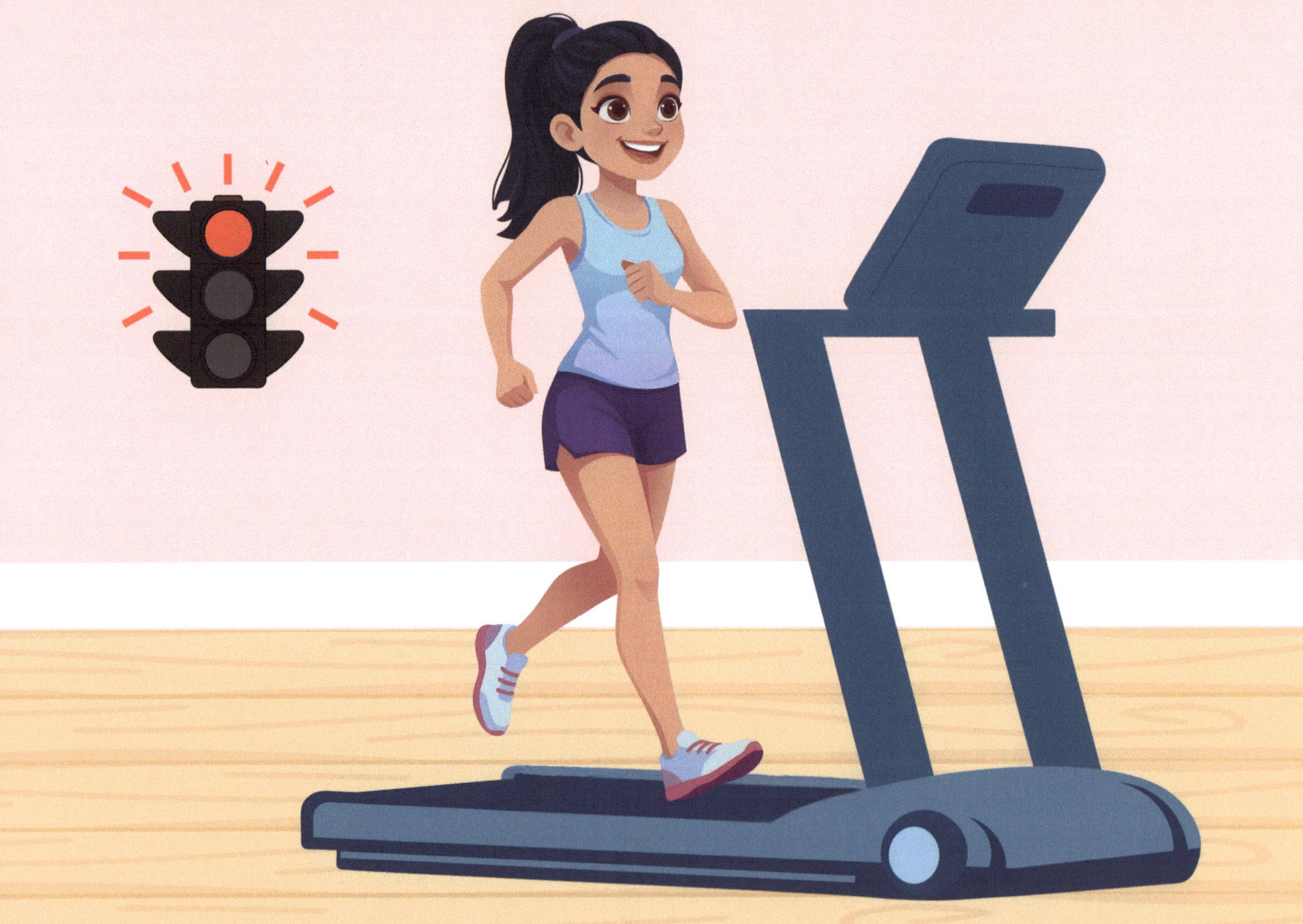

But when she is ready, the light turns to green,
the smoothest transition that she's ever seen.

It softens and opens to let it all go,
no need to rush... just letting life flow.

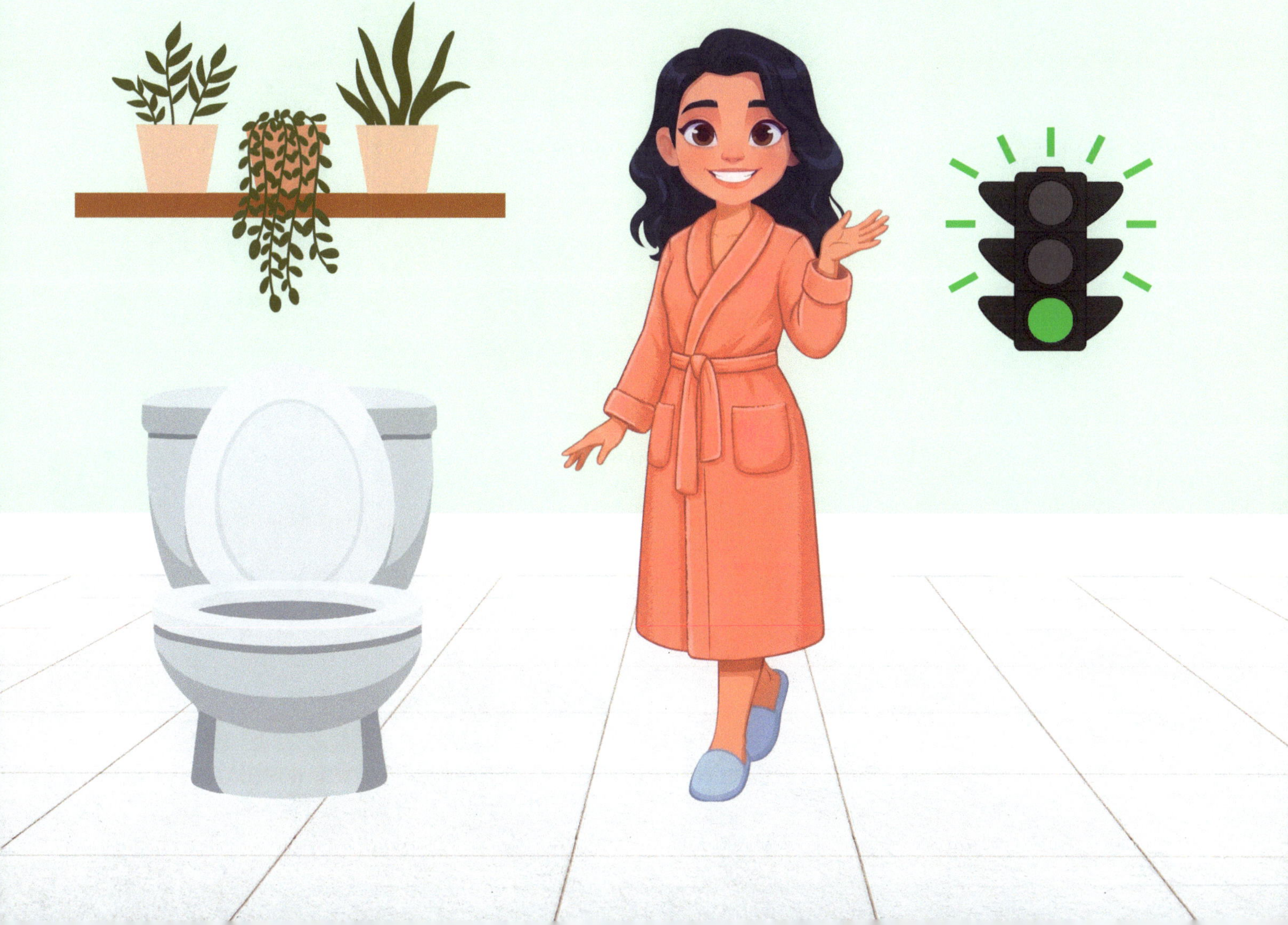

It has a best friend that lives in her chest,
the diaphragm rises and falls without rest.

Like a mirror, they move in a rhythm so fine,
keeping both breath and pressure gently aligned.

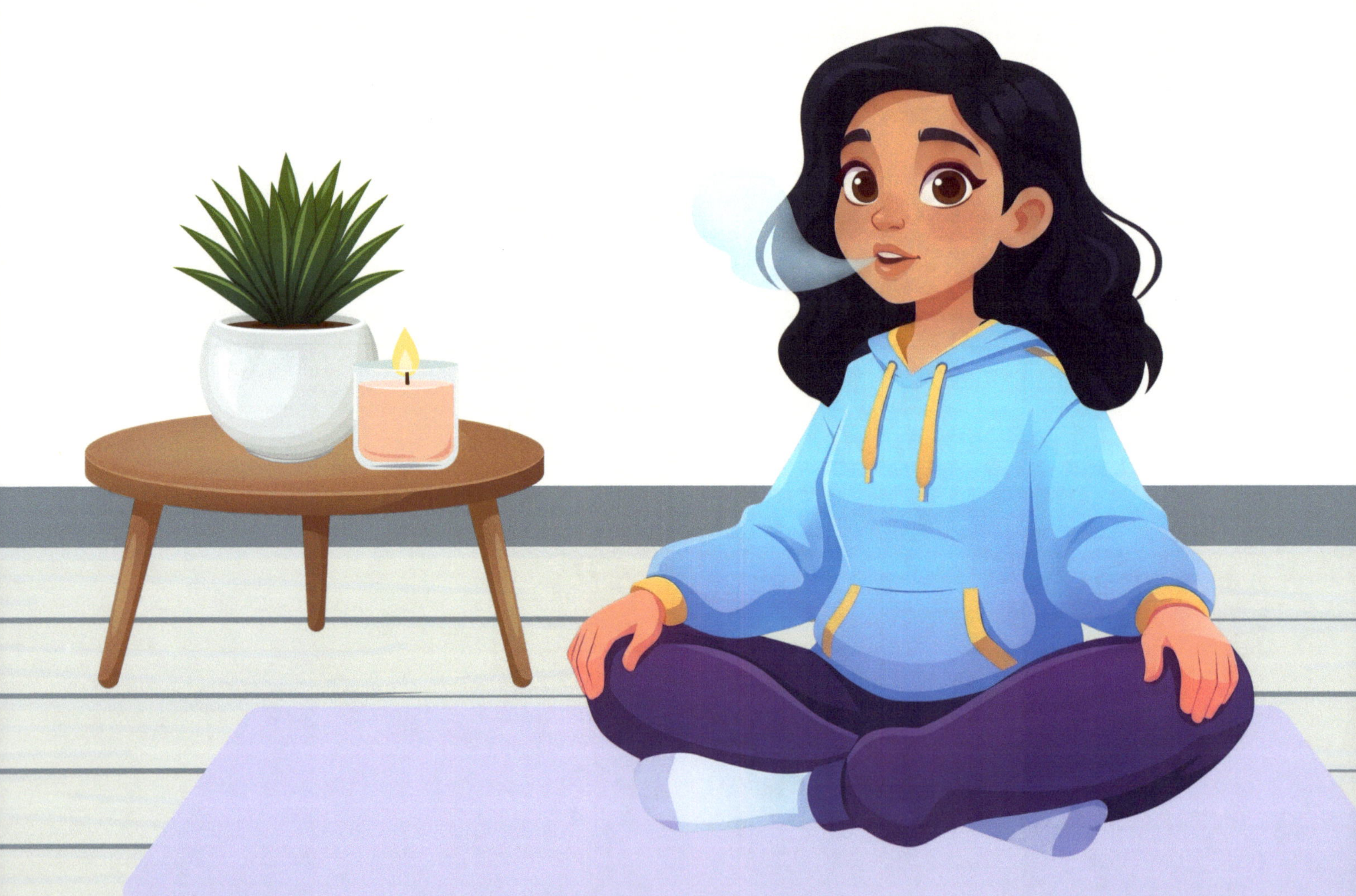

With her deep core muscles,
they form a strong base,
giving her movements
both power and grace.

A balanced foundation
from front to back,
they keep her whole body
steady on track.

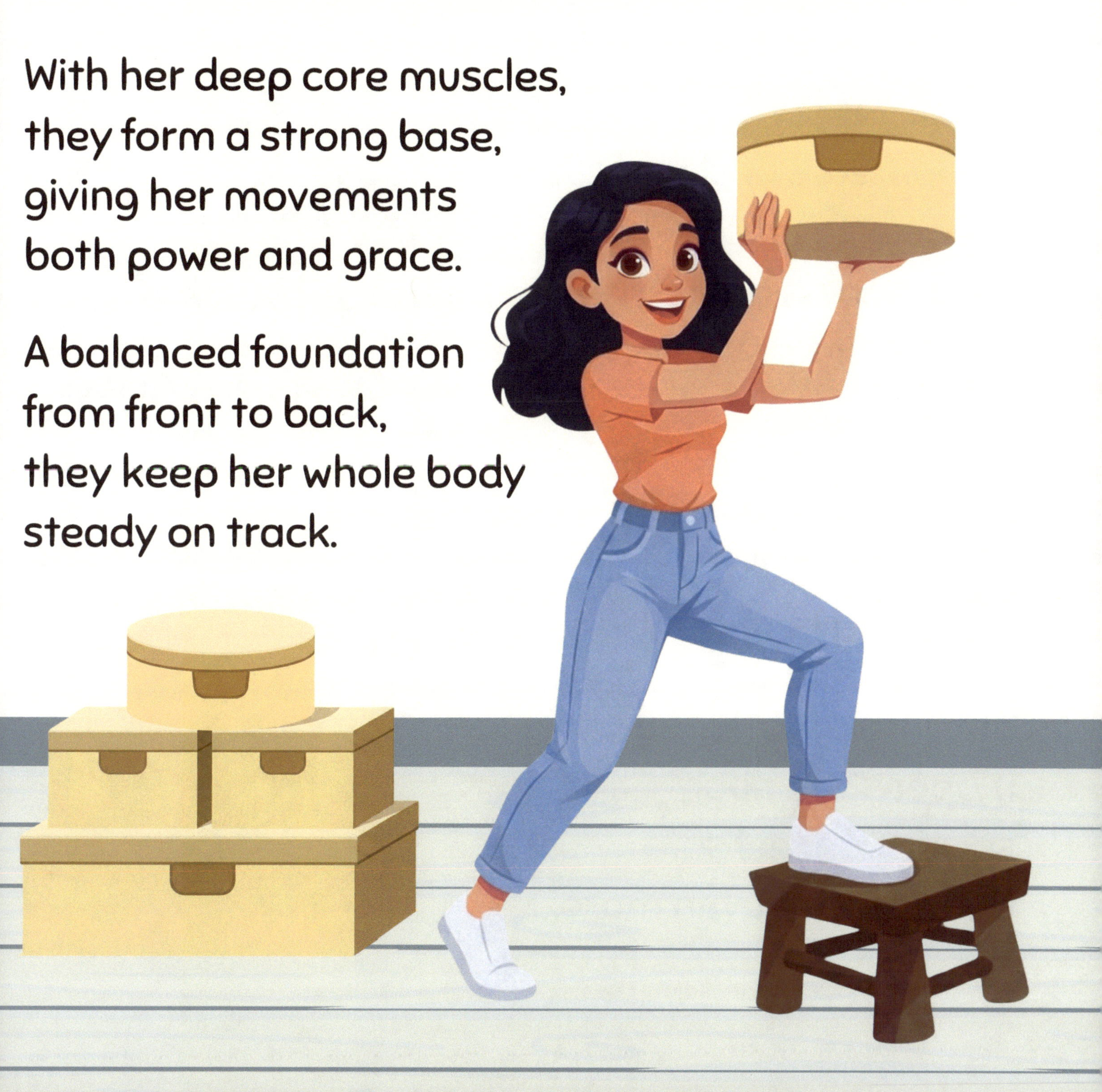

In moments of closeness,
it learns to let go,
softening its hold
to let intimacy flow.

For if it stays guarded,
or tight, or too tense,
it might feel like a wall
or a sturdy defense.

But with breath and patience,
it opens the door,
so she can feel safe
and can love even more.

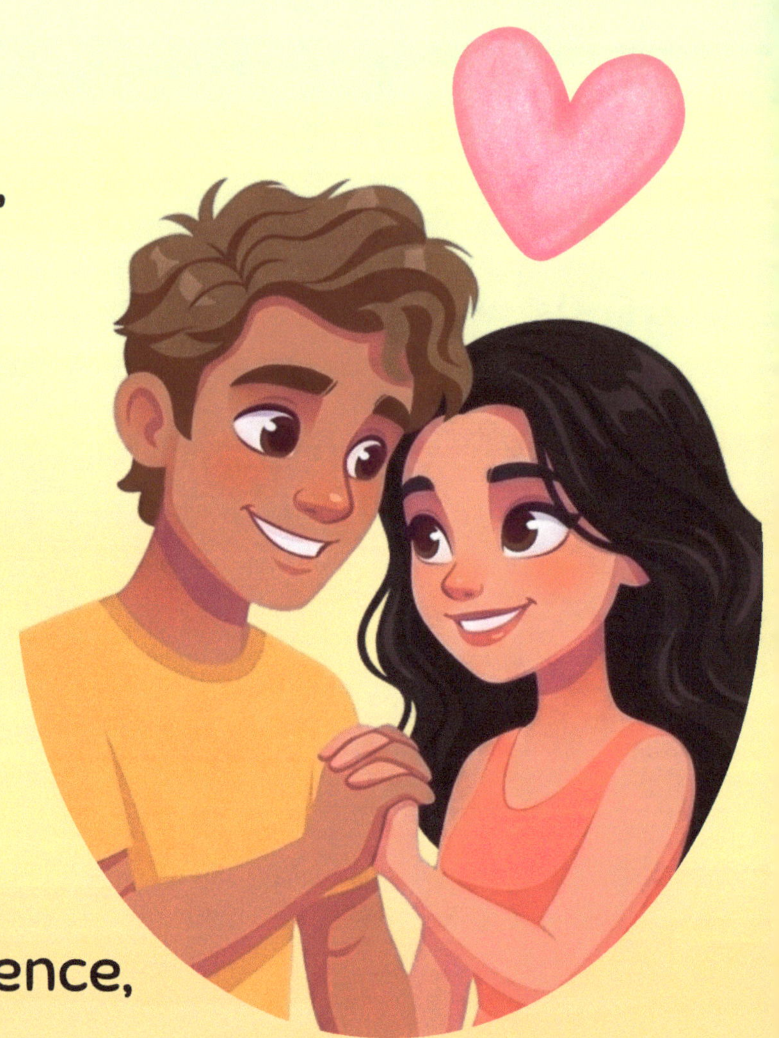

It lifts through pregnancy,
steady and strong,
supporting her baby
all the months long.

To welcome new life,
it prepares for the day,
by softening and stretching
to clear the way.

From holding and lifting
to letting life through,
it's truly amazing what
these muscles can do!

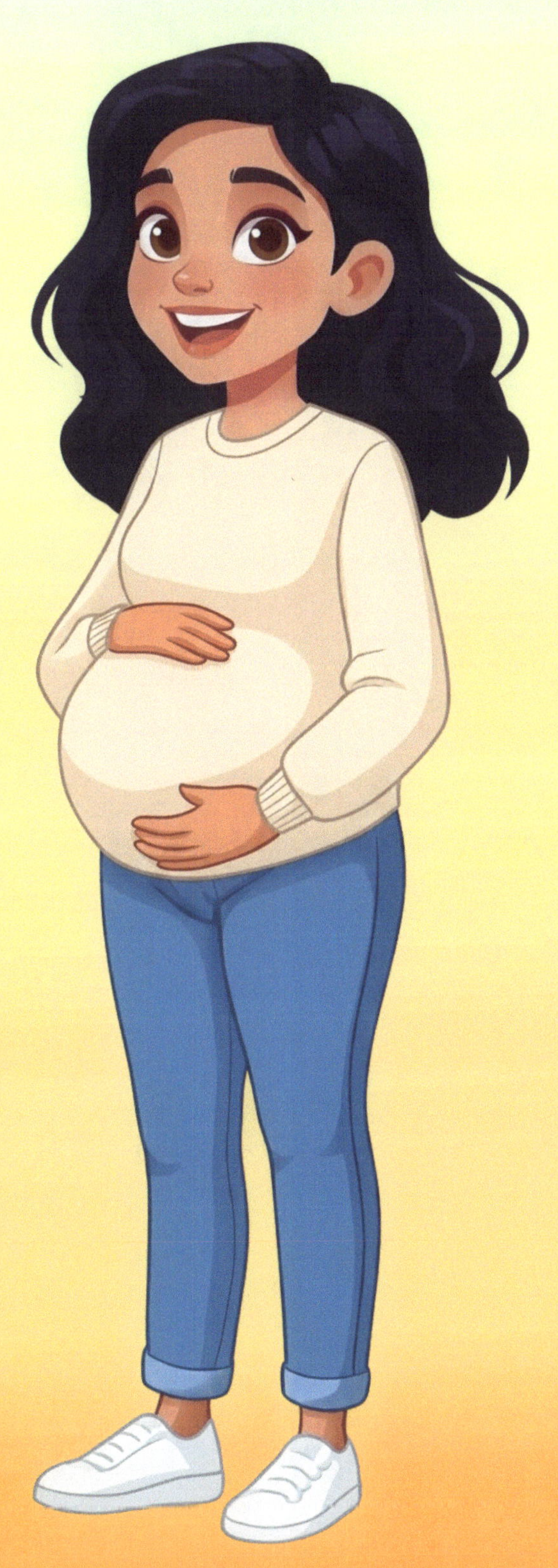

Because it must work through the night and the day,
it can feel overwhelmed in its own quiet way.

Through pregnancy, birth, or seasons of stress,
with aging, high impact, or long days of "yes."

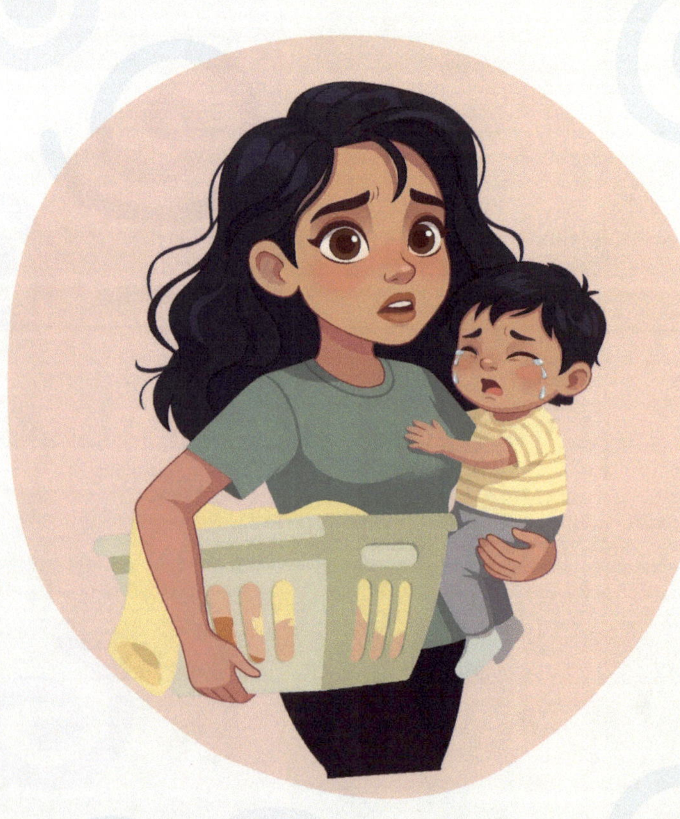

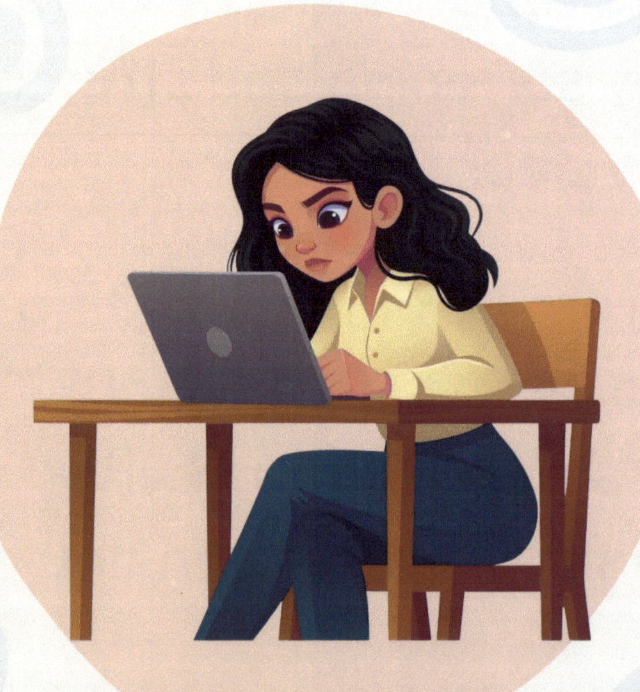

It may whisper through leaking, heaviness, strain,
or speak up with tension, discomfort, or pain.

These signals are cues, it is time to go slow
and listen more closely to what's down below.

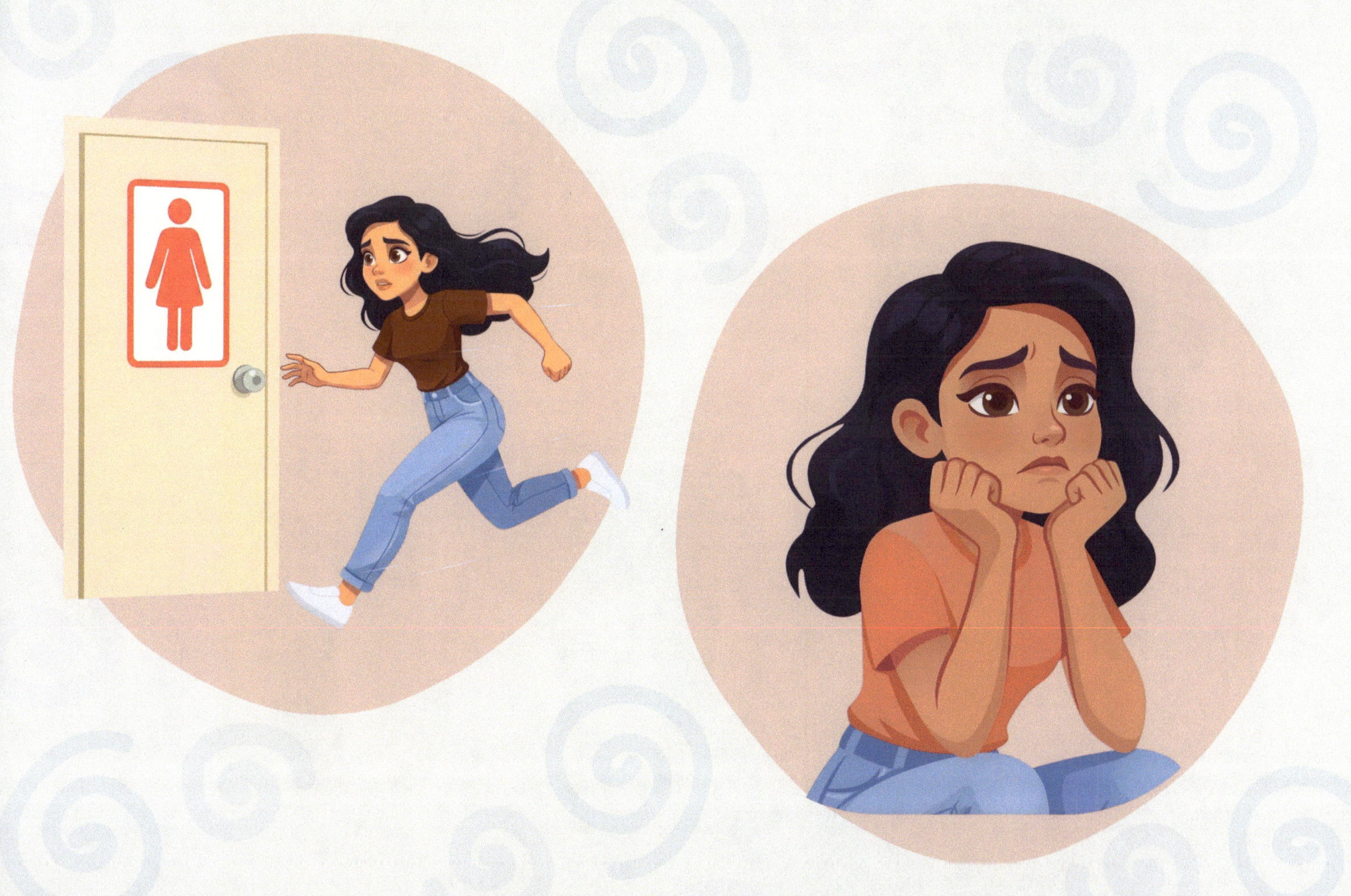

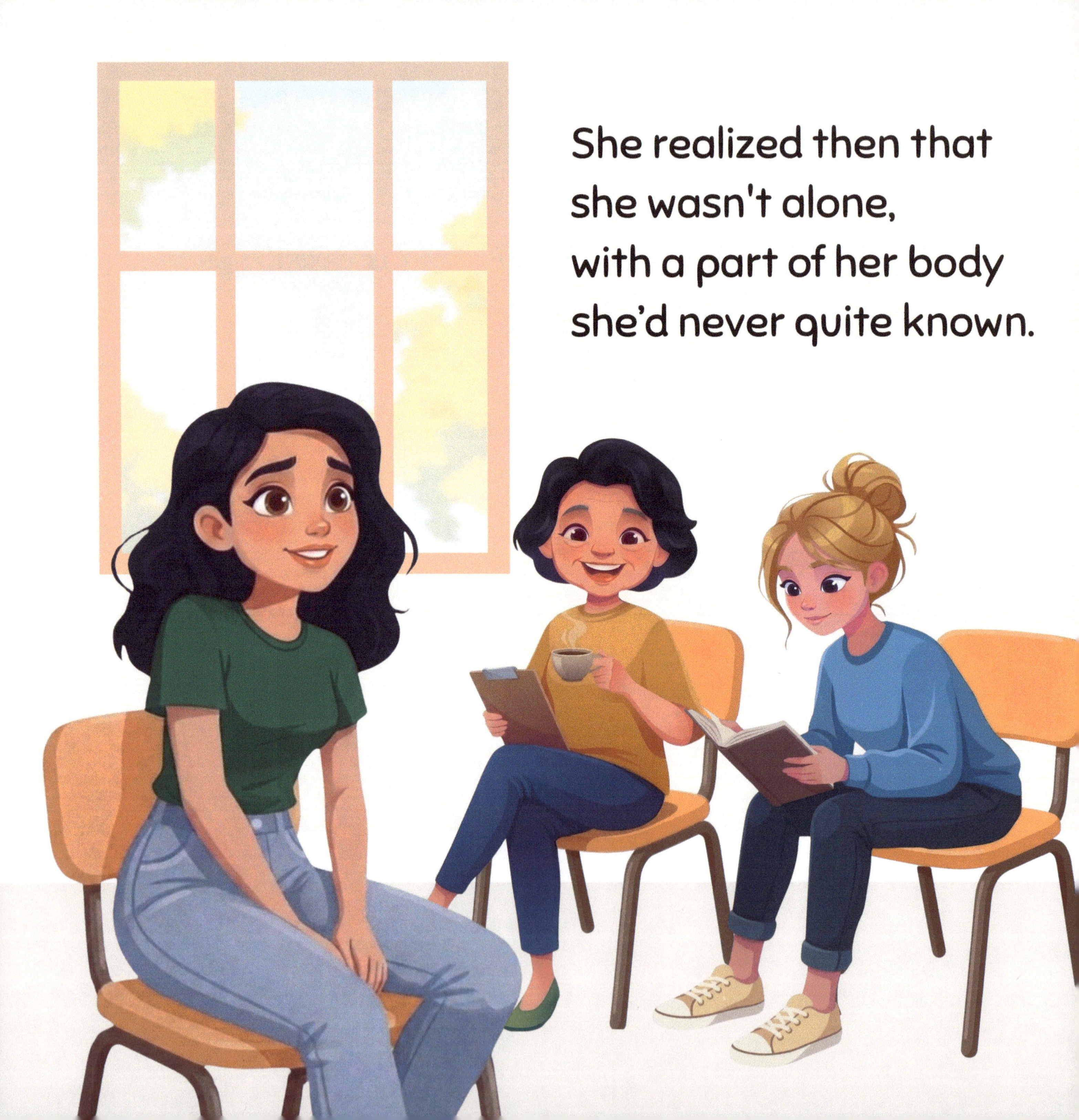

She realized then that
she wasn't alone,
with a part of her body
she'd never quite known.

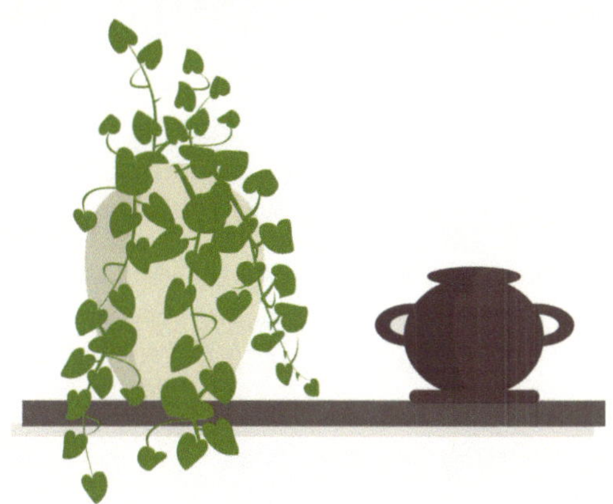

There are experts who guide,
there is no need to fear.
The way back to balance
is finally clear.

A pelvic health pro
helps the rhythm return,
with secrets to share
and new lessons to learn.

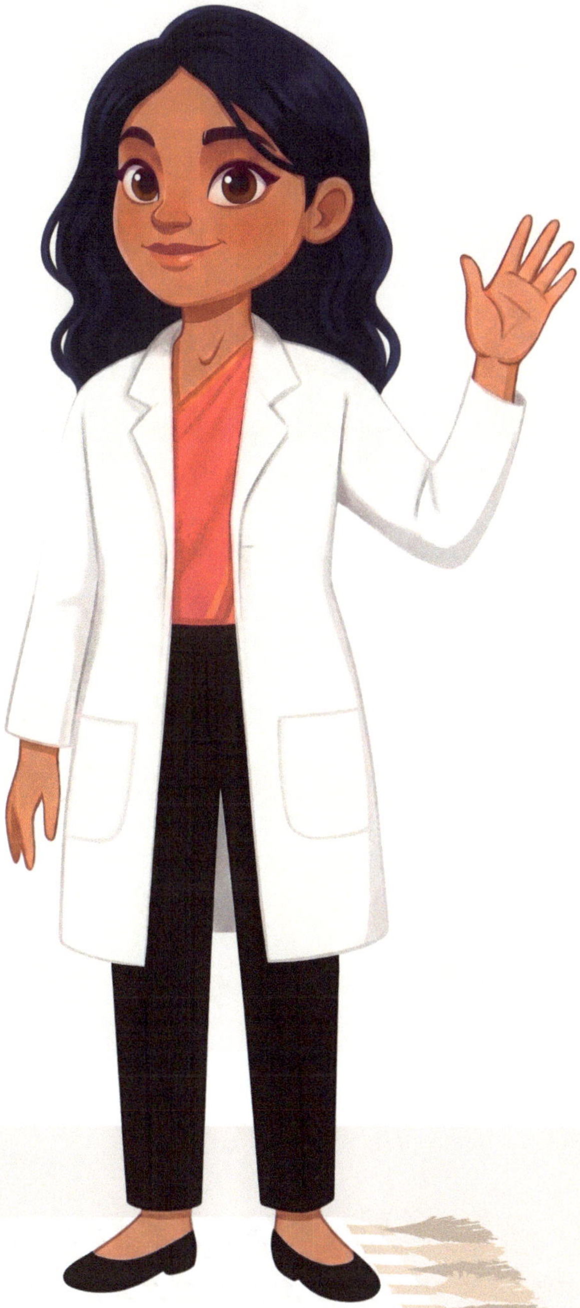

With a thorough assessment
and tools for the task,
they answer the questions
she's wanted to ask.

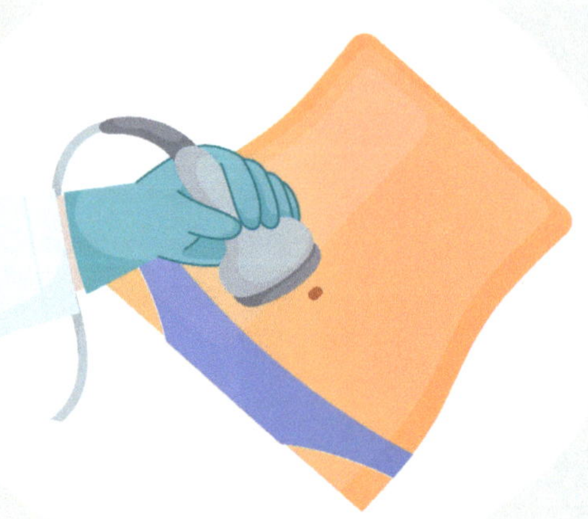

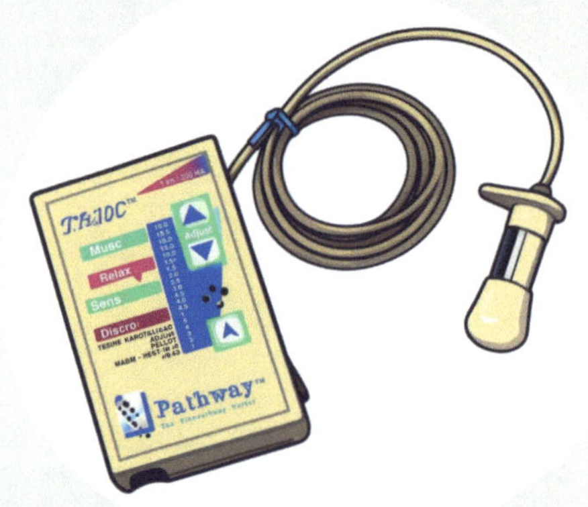

There are sensors and screens
that help guide the release,
and soft pelvic wands that
bring tension to peace.

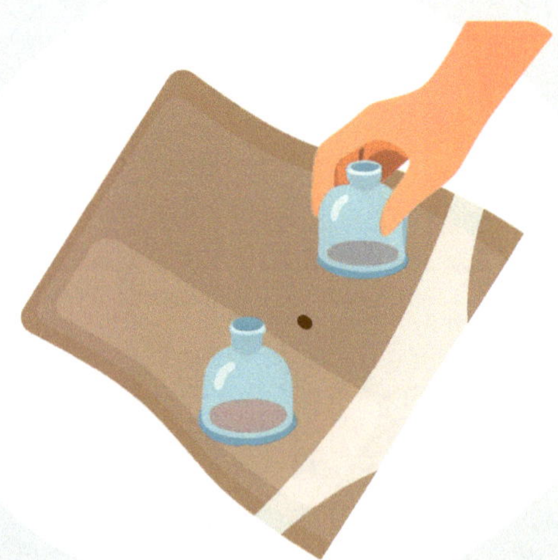

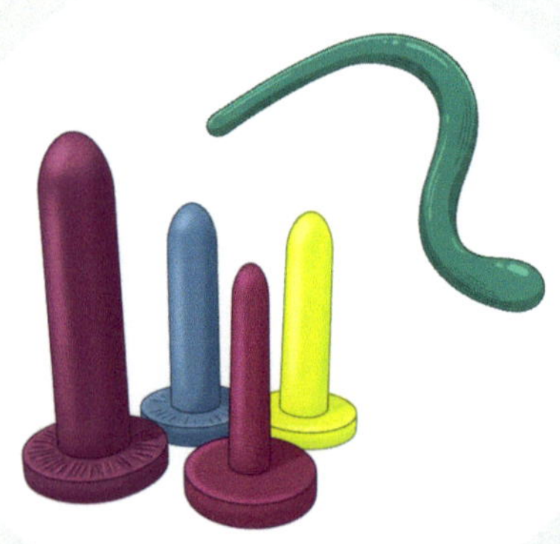

With stretches and gentle, skilled hands that unwind,
they help her body and breath stay aligned.

A well-rounded plan for the strength she will gain,
to move past the leaking, the pressure, the pain.

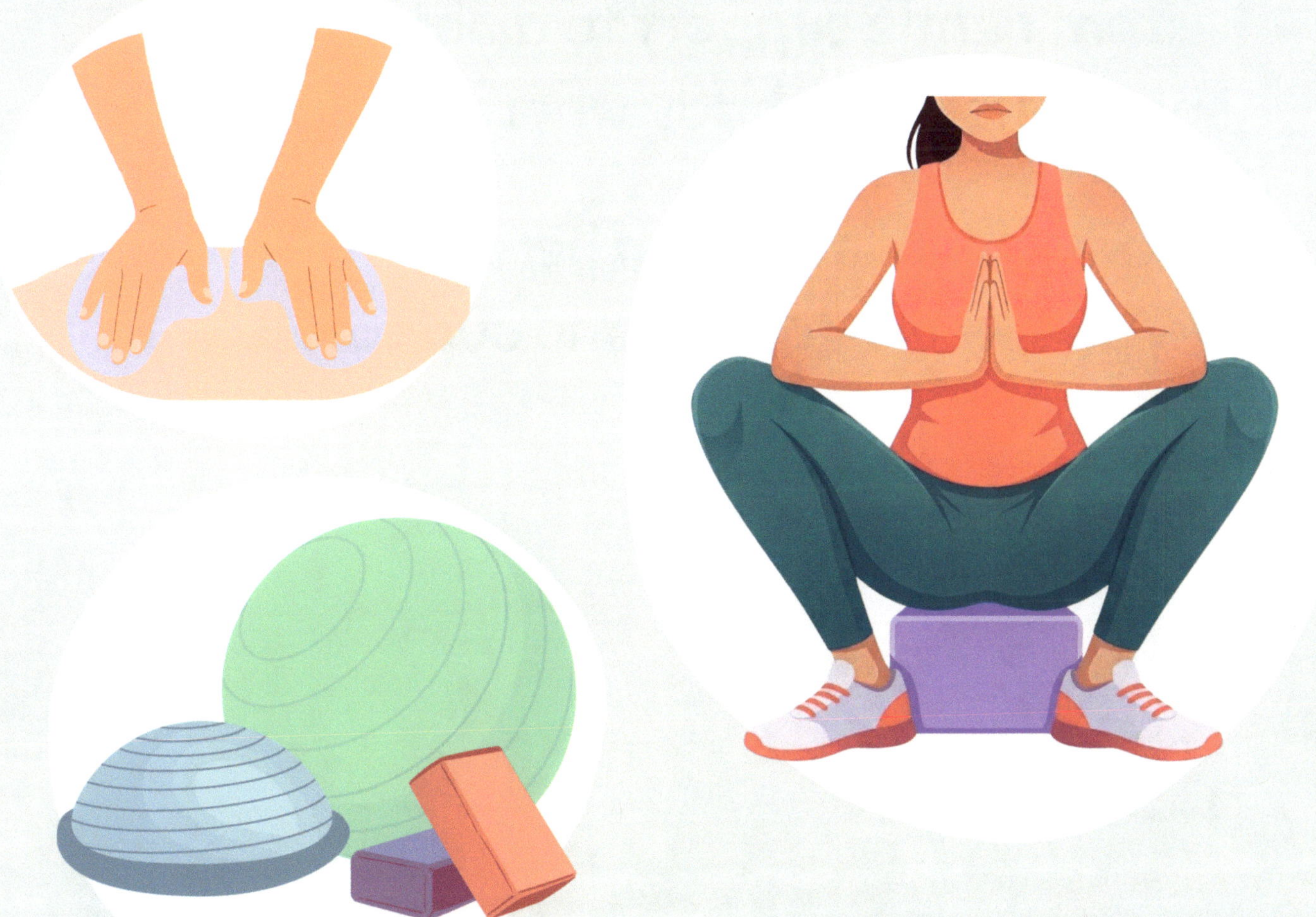

Now, when she laughs, jumps, moves, or lifts,
through every sneeze, and life's little shifts,

from gentle support to a natural flow,
she trusts in her body wherever she goes.

And if something feels off, if her rhythm's not right,
She knows where to turn and support is in sight.

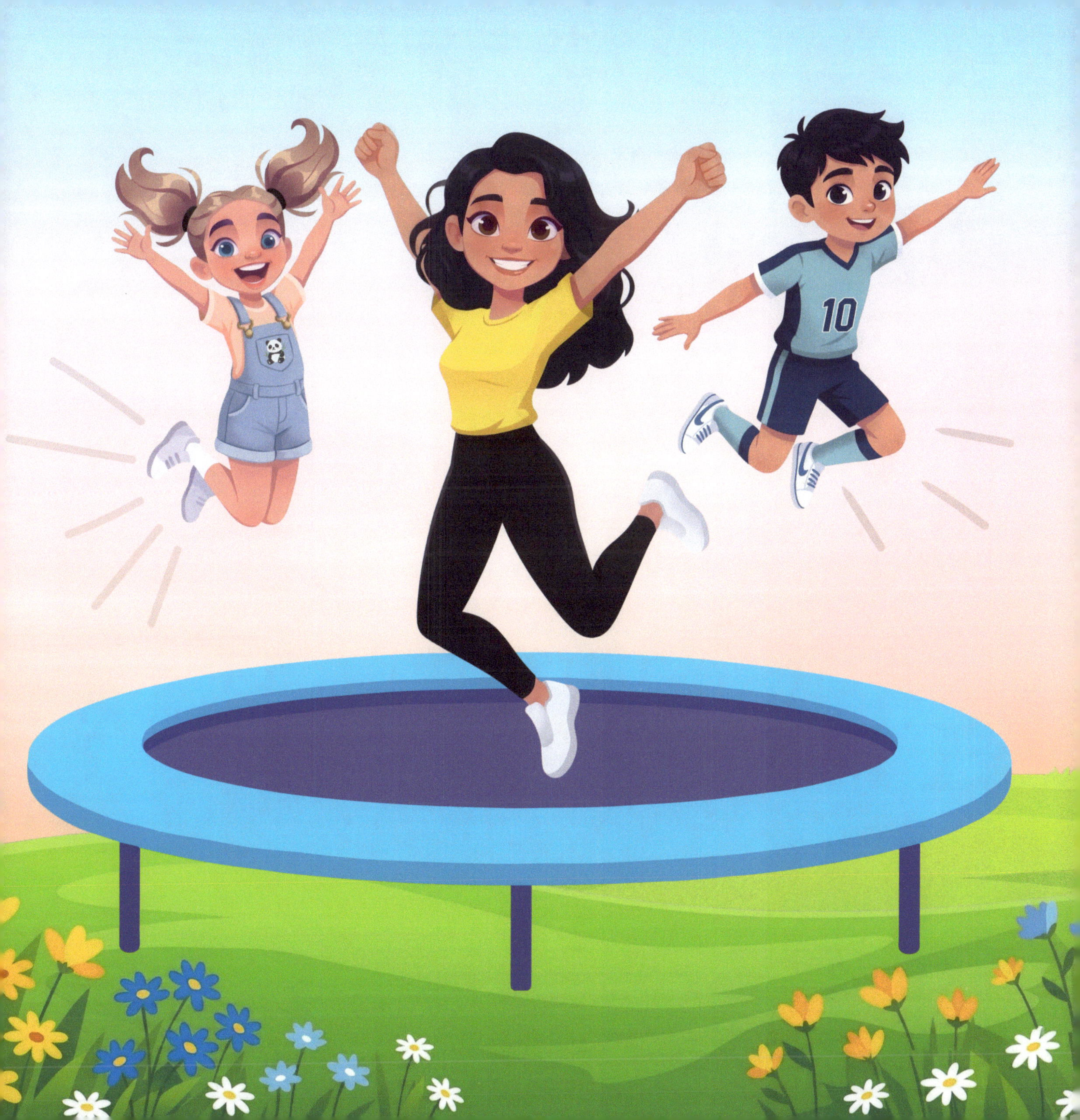

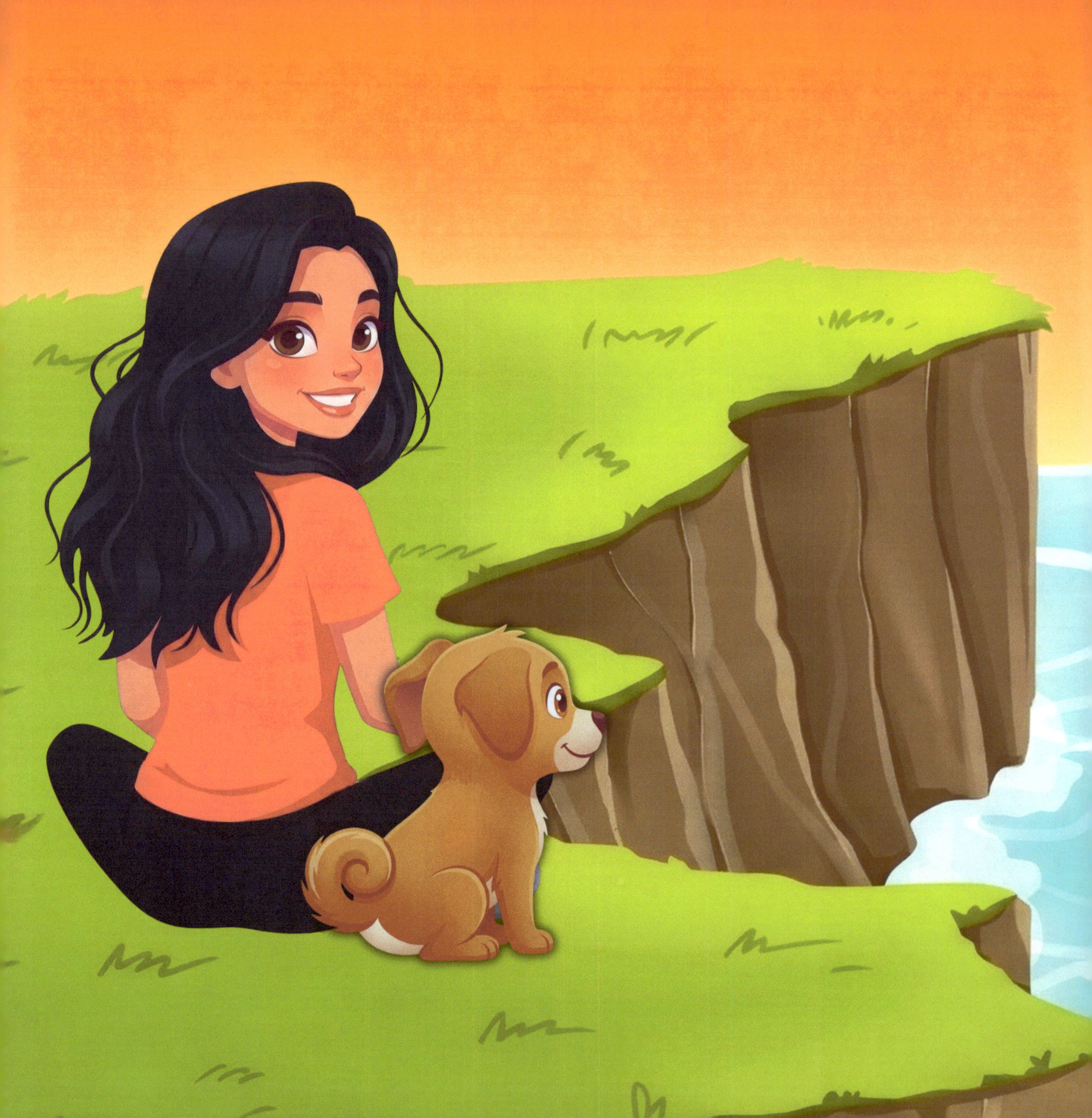

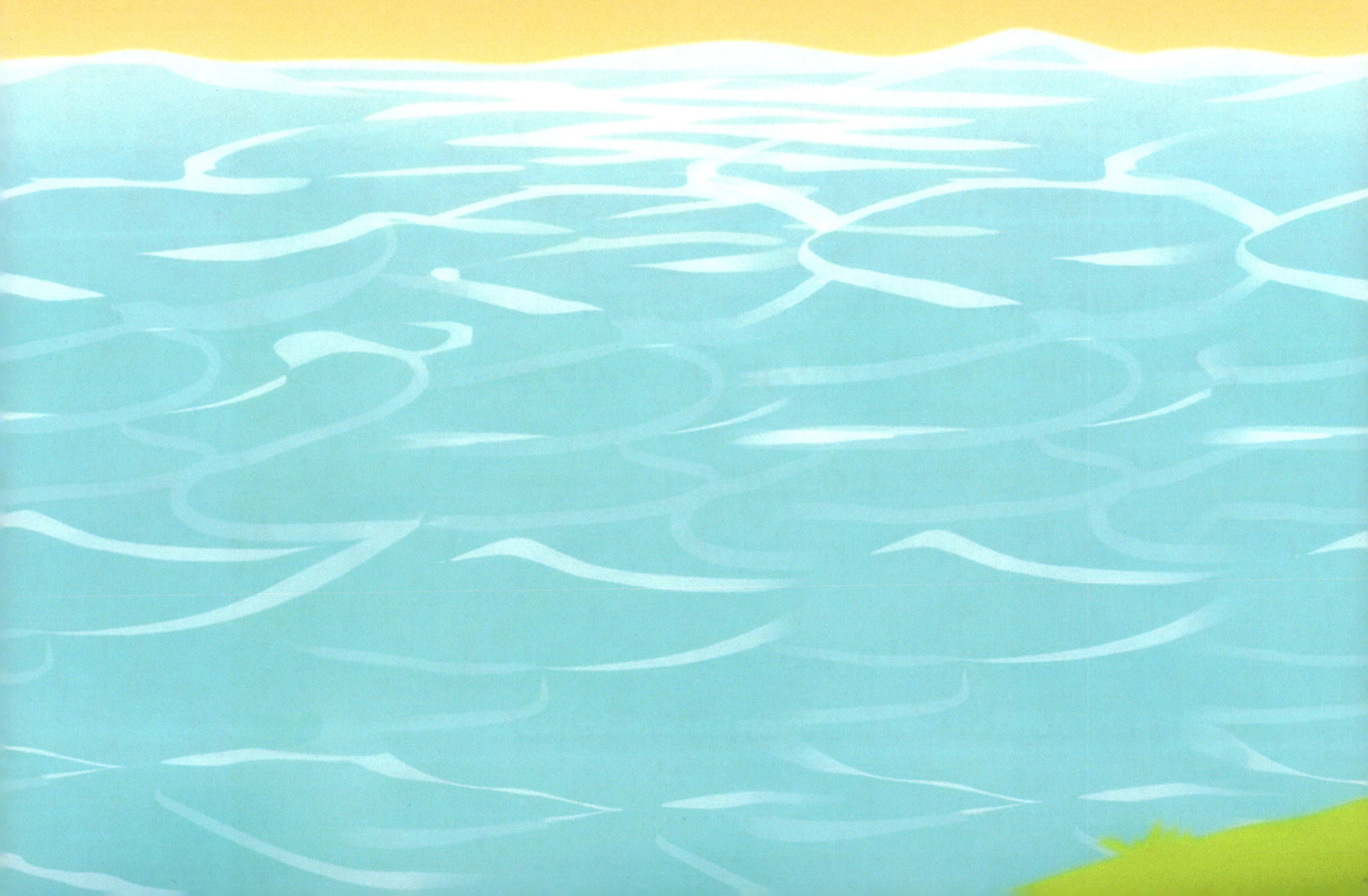

There is joy in her heart for the knowledge she's gained
and pride in the progress she's worked to attain.

For her body is wise, full of beauty and grace...
her pelvic floor now a cherished safe space.

Ways you can care for your pelvic floor

Take A Deep Breath

Find a cozy spot where you feel comfortable.

Place one hand on your belly
and one hand over your heart.

Inhale slowly through your nose,
then exhale slowly through your mouth.

As you breathe in,
feel your belly gently rise.

As you breathe out,
let your body soften and relax.

Gentle Stretching

Try a few stretches that help your hips and pelvis relax. Move slowly. Breathe deeply. Listen to your body.

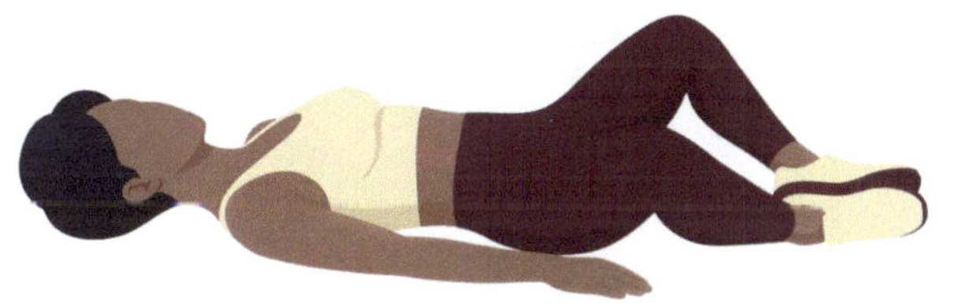

Butterfly Stretch

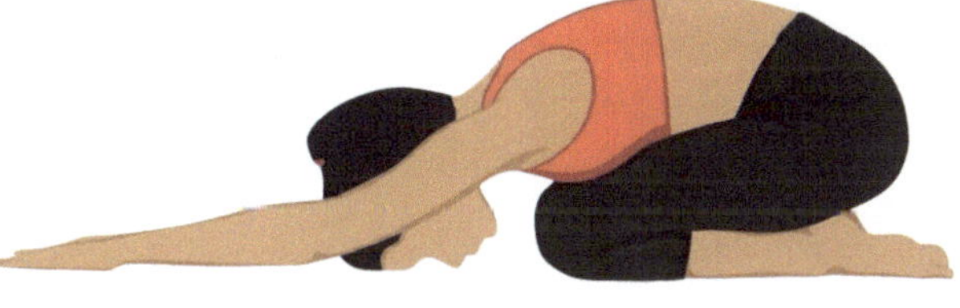

Child's Pose

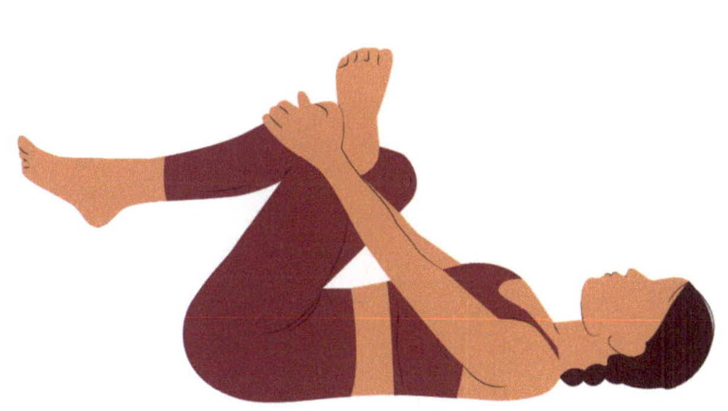

Figure 4 Stretch

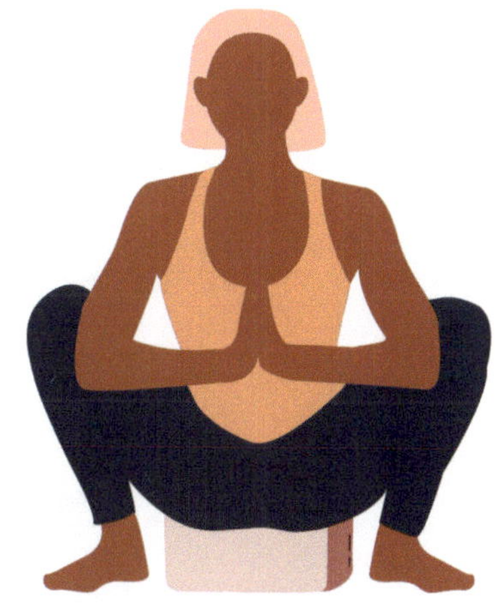

Deep Supported Squat

Build Your Core Foundation

Your pelvic floor works as a team with your core muscles. Strengthen gently and move with intention.

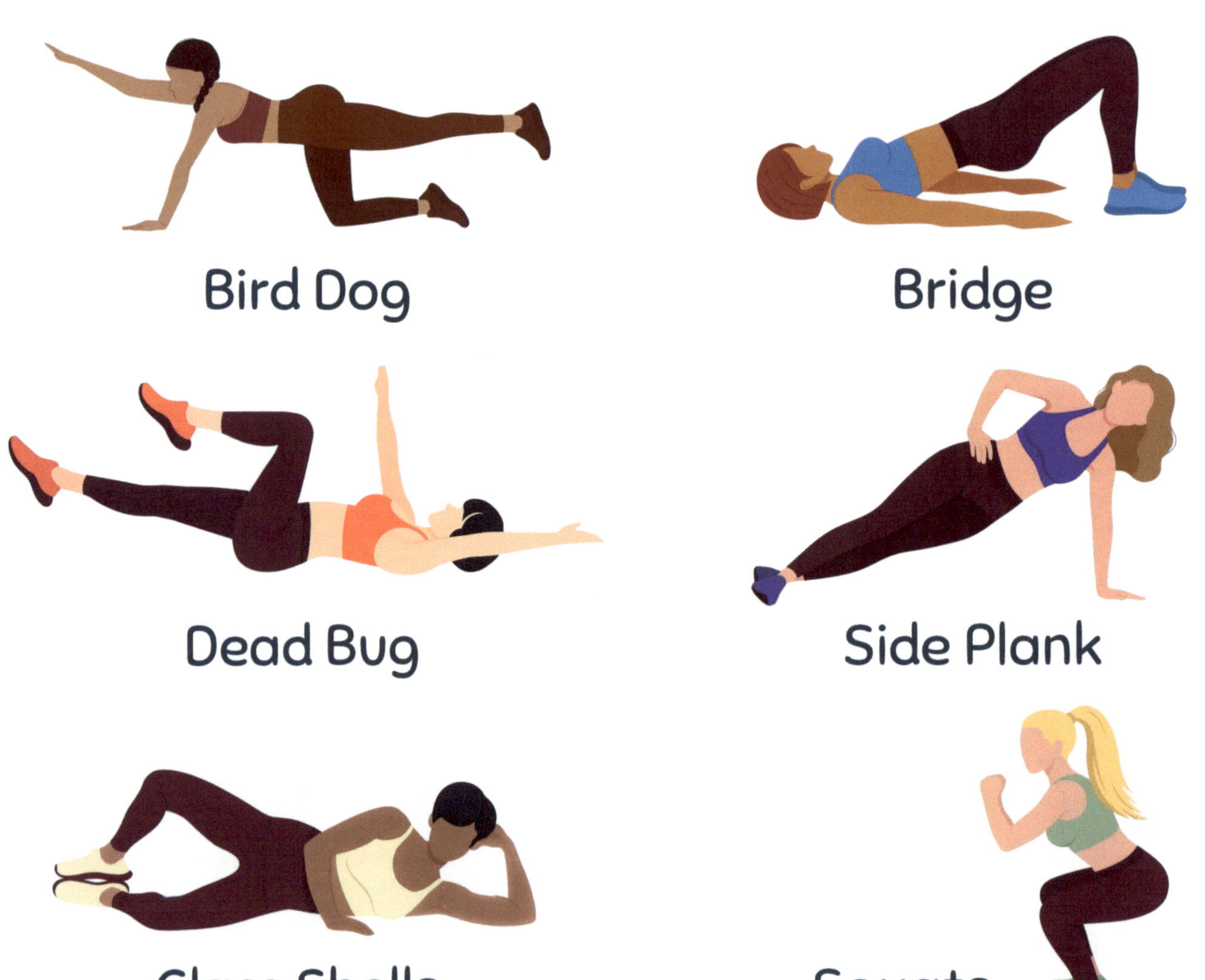

Everyday Pelvic Health Habits

Sip water throughout the day to stay hydrated.

Eat fiber rich foods to support healthy digestion.

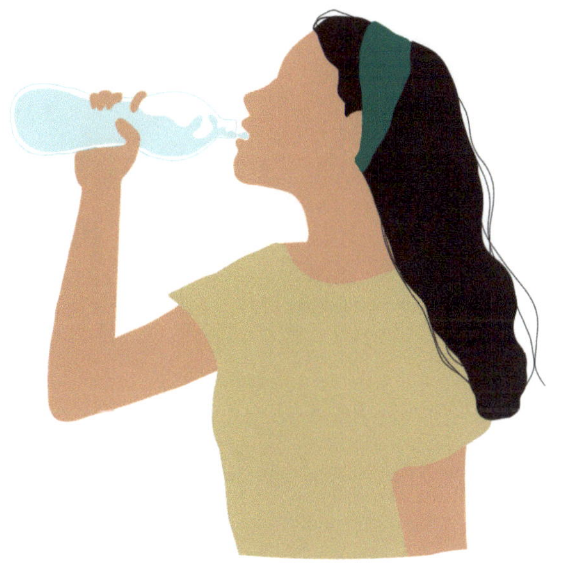

Take your time when using the bathroom and avoid rushing.

Keep your body moving with walking, stretching, and strengthening.

Nurture your body with rest and self-care.

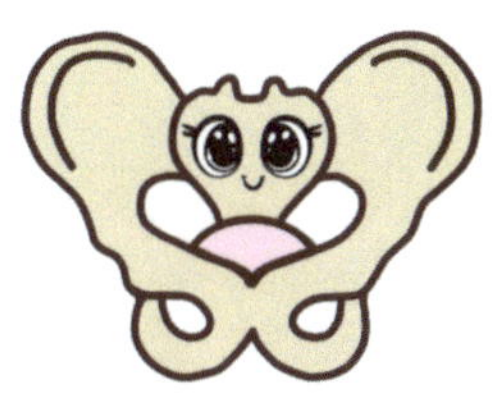

Your Pelvic Floor Thanks You!

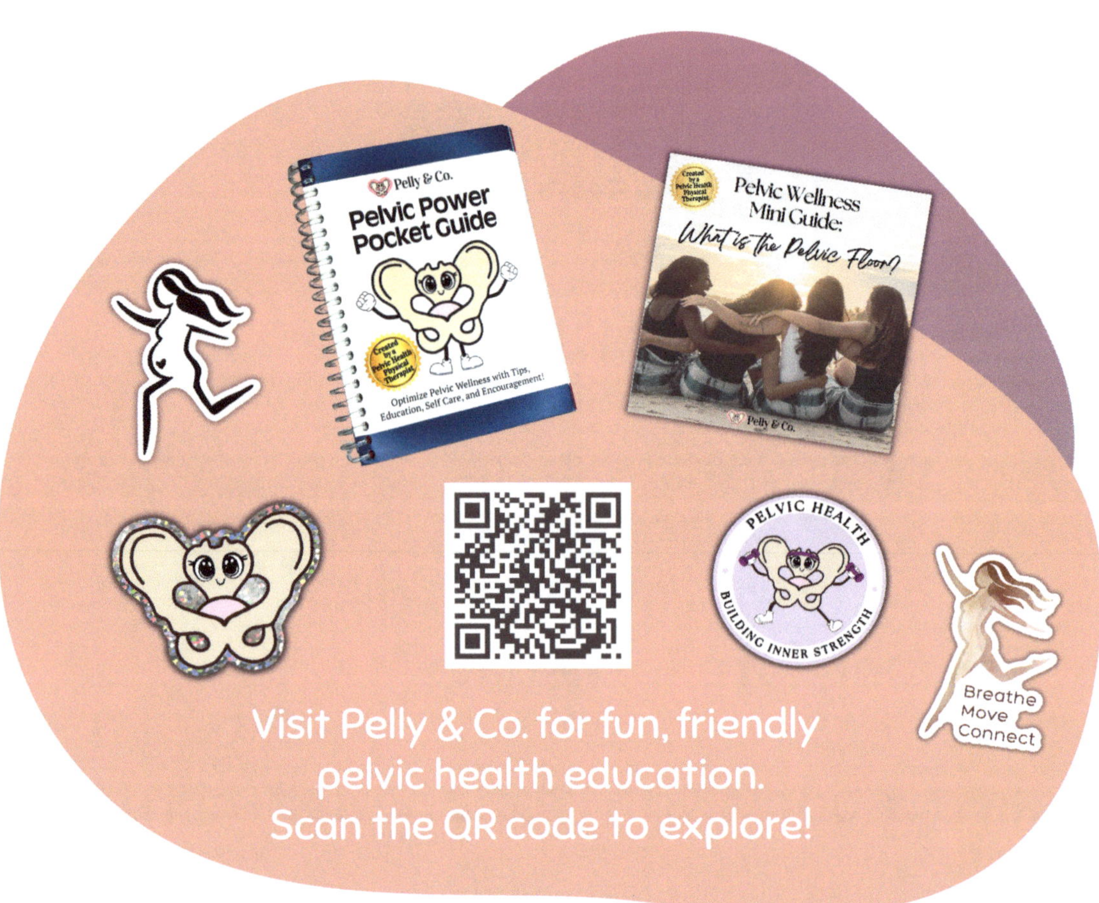
Pelly & Co.
Pelvic Power
Pocket Guide
Created by a Pelvic Health Physical Therapist
Optimize Pelvic Wellness with Tips, Education, Self Care, and Encouragement!
Created by a Pelvic Health Physical Therapist
Pelvic Wellness Mini Guide:
What is the Pelvic Floor?
Pelly & Co.
PELVIC HEALTH
BUILDING INNER STRENGTH
Breathe
Move
Connect
Visit Pelly & Co. for fun, friendly pelvic health education.
Scan the QR code to explore!

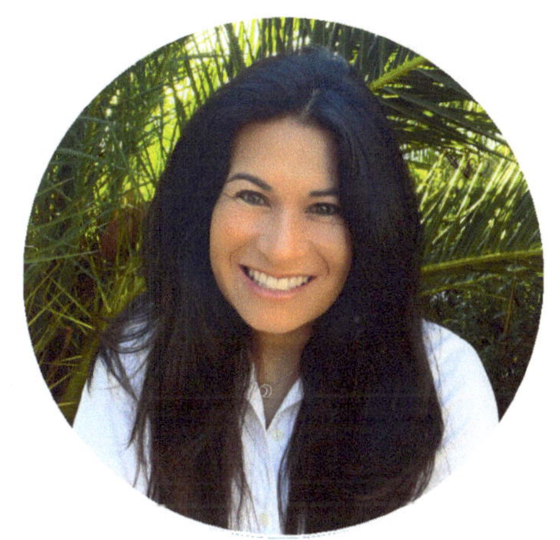

About the Author

Michelle B. Loureiro is a Pelvic Health Physical Therapist dedicated to helping women understand and care for their bodies with confidence.

After years of hearing the phrase, "I wish I'd known this sooner," she was inspired to share pelvic health knowledge in ways that are simple, approachable, and empowering. She is the creator of Pelly & Co., a playful educational brand that helps make learning about pelvic health fun and supportive.

Michelle lives in Southern California, where she enjoys hiking, spending time with her family, and taking her dog to the beach.